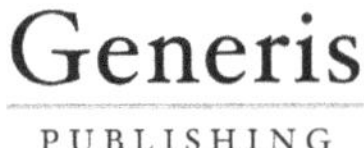
Generis
PUBLISHING

AF579455

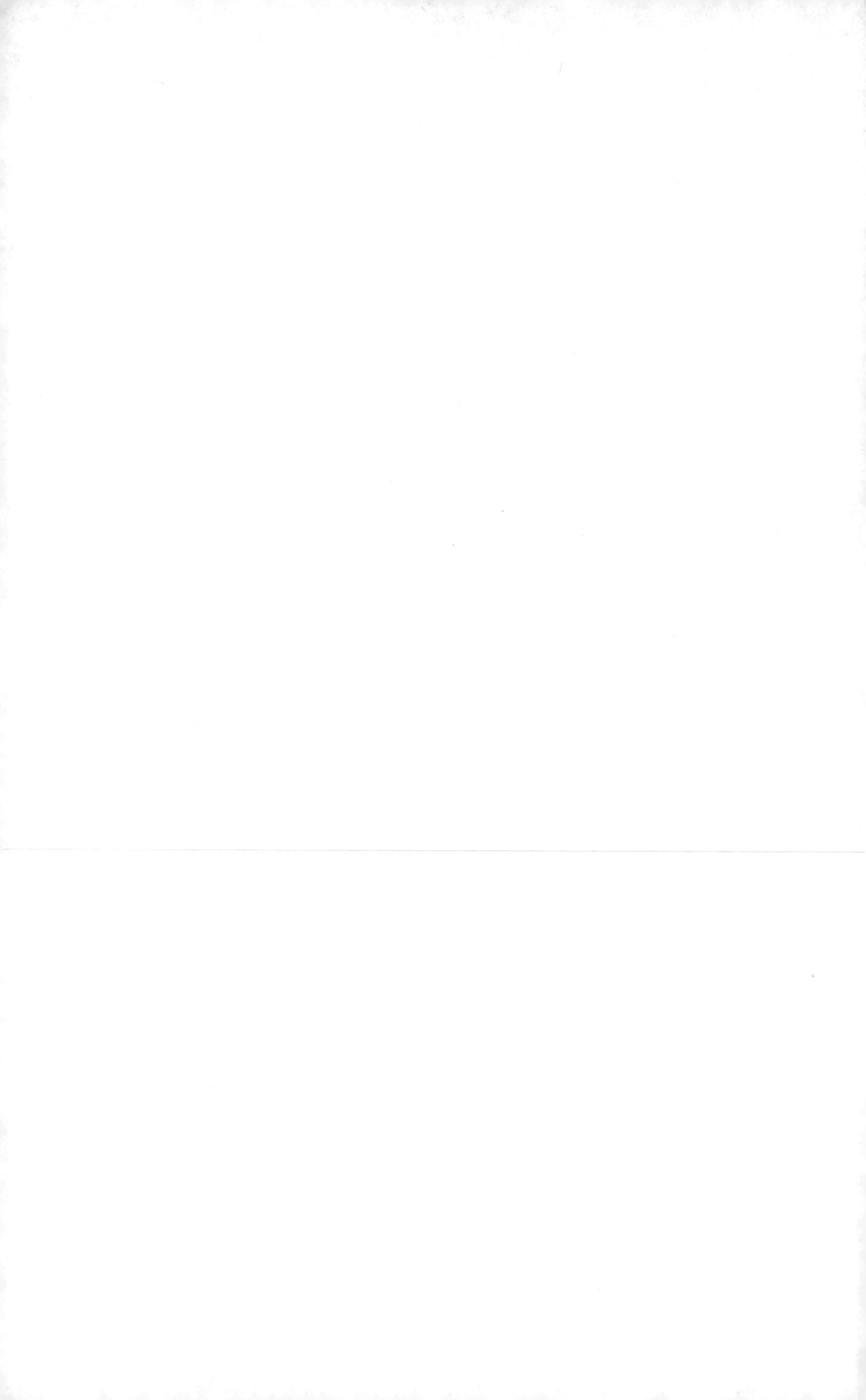

Together, without... discrimination!

Applied-thematic guide

Maria Dorina Pașca

Title: **Together, without... discrimination!**

Applied-thematic guide

ISBN: 979-8-89248-599-9

Author: Maria Dorina Paşca

Cover image: www.pixabay.com

Publisher: Generis Publishing
Online orders: www.generis-publishing.com
Contact email: info@generis-publishing.com

Maria Dorina Pașca

Together, without...

discrimination!

(Applied-thematic guide)

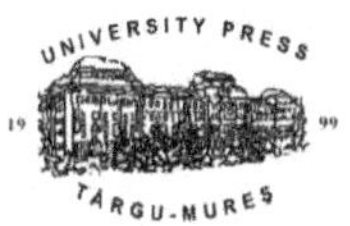

2018

Author: Maria Dorina Paşca

Translation: Roxana- Maria Iagăr

Referees: Ceană Daniela - Edith

Csibi Șandor

Publisher University Press is recognized by The National Council for Scientific Research in Higher Education (CNCSIS) - Cod 210.

Typewriting:
Printing: The center of Copy and Multimedia- University Press Targu Mureș, 2018

CIP description of the National Library of Romania Maria Dorina Pașca

Together... without discrimination!! / Maria Dorina Paşca; (Applied-thematic guide). - Targu Mureş: University Press, 2018

Bibliography ISBN 978-973-169-522-8

The translation was made with permission of the author in the current year, 2024 (Roxana-Maria Iagăr)

Contents

About

Applied- thematic guide, Together, without... discrimination! is the logistic ways through which the knowledge about the characteristics of vulnerable groups in the health system, implemented through the elements of ethics and non-discrimination, is deepened.

Practical concept, as a landmark in recognizing, but also solving problems, the applied-thematic guide, together without...discrimination! Complete in personal way, attractive, pleasant, interesting, intelligent tolerant and creative, the theoretic part of knowledge acquired in this cognitive field of ethics and non-discrimination.

Being a working tool, the applied- thematic guide ***Together, without... discrimination***, creates the opportunity for the student to get involved directly, through their own opinions, concepts and examples, their life experience is welcomed, bringing their personality element through new cognitive, instructive- educational identities and more.

In this context, the applied- thematic guide, ***Together, without... discrimination!*** responds constructively and creatively to an educational requirement, starting from the idea of equality and having as motto: "respect, to be respected"

Conf.univ.dr.psih.

Maria Dorina Pașca

A) Concepts

1.The vulnerable group is formed by:

a) Children (why?)

b) Pregnant women (why?)

c) Elders (Why?)

d) Mentally ill (Why?)

2. The 10 rules on cultural interference in medical practice are:

1) Cultural identification:

Applications:

- Find a person from the group
- Work in teams
- Learn the basic elements of patient's culture

2) Communication method:

Applications:

- Seeking to find your own channel and personal communication
- Let them to communicate
- Find a translator in extreme cases

3) Language barrier

Applications:

- identify the verbal and non-verbal language barriers
- use the non-verbal information in verbal

- if you know the patient's language, it's important to connect what you say to how you say

4) Understanding:

Applications:

- let your patient speak
- understand the mechanism of their minds and language
- speak understandable by the patient

5) Beliefs and values involved:

Applications:

- don't make value judgments without cover
- accept the opinion of the others

6) Trust

Applications:

- Prove you're trustworthy by what you do
- Trust helps the prognosis of the disease
- Your activity is, the life card…. of trust"

7) Healing

Applications:

-Don't promise the impossible

-Make sure that recovery is plausible/ truthful

-Respond to all requesting regarding the patient recovered

8) The diet

Applications:

- Team up with your nutritionist
- Know the traditions and eating habits of the patient

9) Evaluation

Applications:

- to be done with responsibility and honesty

- attention to emotional involvement

- know cultural differences

10) Medical team's subjectivism:

- don't forget you took an oath
- do not make differences of any rank
- we are equals and not… different

3. **Discrimination** means treating a person less favorably because of:

- Rase
- Ethnicity
- Nationality
- Disability
- Religion
- Age
- Sexual orientation, as well as other criteria prohibited by law

Example

- Refuse to receive family doctor's list, a patient or to
- provide medical assistance because it is of Roma ethnicity gypsy
- Applications: -discover the message from Hippocrates' oath (extracted):

"I swear! I will endure the care of the sick for their benefit, as much as my powers and my mind will help me, and I will avoid doing them any harm and injustice"

Discrimination represents the different treatment of a person due to his belonging to a particular group.

Applications:

a) The message in the Prayer of Maimonides (fragment) is:

"I beg you, do not let me deviate from the noble labor of helping my fellow men.

Forgive me and strengthen my powers of body and mind

so that I may be ever ready to help both the rich and the poors, the good and the bad, those who love and those who hate and let me see in the sickest of men..."

b) Find three situations regarding discrimination in the health system:

1.

2.

3.

4.Vulnerability

- It's a modern concept that tends to take the place of the concept of endogenous determinism (Lăzărescu M-1994)
- It's a catalyst that amplifies the effect of a triggering agent whether it is a major event or serious life difficulty, and which is only effective in relation to them. (Tudose FI 2003)

Applications:

a) I felt vulnerable/ when

b) for me to be vulnerable/ means and represent

c) Find the elements that define the vulnerabilities of the health system:

1.

2.

3.

5. **Prejudice** refers to preconceived opinions that someone has about something, someone without direct knowledge of the facts.

Applications:

a) Explains the message, the statement: “who is not with us, is against us”.

b) True or false:

If you are from the country, are you?

- Old and stupid/ young and smart?
- The gypsy is always the thief?
- If you stay in the first bench, are you in, the bench of donkeys?

c) Find situations related to prejudices in the health system.

1.

2.

3.

6. **The stereotype** understood as a preconceived and oversimplified notion of the typical characteristics of a person or group.

Applications

a) The following stereotypes are true or false: (motivates)

- All teachers are women

- All people on the streets are alcoholics

- All gypsies are criminals

b) creates 1-2 stereotypes:

1.

2.

b) Find stereotypes in health system:

1.

2.

3.

7. Equality is a principle according to which all people and all states or nations recognize the same rights and imposed the same duties, as provided for by the rule of law.

Applications:

a) For me, to be equal to someone, something, is:

b) Explains the message of the quotations:

“Under all aspects, so treat yourself fellows, as you would like to treat yourself, they”

“Any you would like to make someone for you do them and you are just.”

c) -Find equality situations or not, in the health system

1.

2.

3.

8. The right to health is an inclusive right that implies freedoms comprising benefits and excluding discrimination

Applications

a) For me, the right to health is

b) Explains the message of the statement: “the human is being and not an object”

c) Find times when the right to. Health in the health system was violated/ not respected? Understood, was respected.

1.

2.

3.

B) Thematic applications

1. Complete the sentences…

1. I feel discriminated/ when:

Why?

2. I feel vulnerable when:

Why?

3. I have prejudiced when:

Why?

4. I feel in minority when:

Why?

5. I'm excluded when:

Why?

6. I'm tolerant when:

Why?

7. I accept respective situation when:

Why?

8. I feel equal to you when:

Why?

2. Continue the sentence…

Being different from others in

a) Family

b) Hospital

c) Community

For me, means

a)

b)

c)

You must choose between two groups:

- One with plus
- Another with minus

Which one do you choose? Which one do you report to?

Why?

Do you feel discriminated if some are standing and others sitting on chairs? How do you perceive this fact?

If yes, why?

If not, why?

Do you know yourself enough? Have you ever been vulnerable/ have you?

If yes, when?

If not, why?

Do you know any words that give life? Do you use them?

If yes, which and why?

If not, why?

Do you mind if someone addresses you with an appellation that later becomes a nickname?

If yes, which and why?

If not, why?

Do you accept being criticized for no reason? How do you react?

If yes, when and why?

If not, why?

Do you accept being praised when you deserve it?

If yes, why?

If not, why?

Compose an exercise-game, according to the previous models:

3. Find the message…

"No matter how you are feeling, get up every morning and prepare to let your light shine forth."

(Paulo Coelho, 2012)

"God, grant me the serenity to change the things I can't change, the courage to change the things I can change and the wisdom to see the difference."

(Prayer of serenity- Paşca MD 2008)

The worst disease is loneliness.

Hospital food tastes like loneliness.

4. Your opinion, it matters…

In a salon is admitted a homeless and during his stay, the patients find out. How do you react if the element discrimination appears?

In the waiting room of the medical office, there is a family of gypsies who make noise and bother. What are you doing?

How do you react?

In the corridors of the hospital, not observing the visiting schedule, a family of gypsies appears, what do you do? How do you react?

When you're on guard, an infected patient with HIV comes to you and tells you this (he/she informs you) only at the end of the medical consultation. How do you react and how do you solve the problem?

On guard, a patient who says he is infected with HIV is brought. What are you doing?

Does it bother you that during the consultation, the patient talks about God? What are you doing? How do you react?

On guard is brought a mother with her child, minor, physically assaulted (beaten). What are you doing?

You're just solving the medical problem? Or are you trying to get socially involved? (social care, child protection, police)

The patient refuses to receive blood, which is vital to saving his/ her life, arguing that religion does not allow him/ her. What are you doing?

A patient provokes you by giving you money for the medical act you undertake. Do you receive them?

A member of the family who is hospitalized offers you money for the medical intervention performed. How do you react?

The patient refuses to be consulted by a female doctor. Refuse the consultation? How do you react? Why?

The patient refuses the consultation to be performed by a male doctor, asking for a female doctor. You accept? How do you react? What are you doing?

At the hospital gate, only the doorman asks you for the entrance ticket, the others do not. How are you feeling?

What are you doing?

You are a doctor and the nurse refuses to work with you.

Do you ask yourself, why?

You don't respect the consultation schedule displayed on the door of your office and the patients are dissatisfied. Do you mind? Affects you? Why?

You are drawn to the indecent outfit that you approach as a medical professional. How do you react? Why?

A patient's family reapproaches you for the medical fault. Does it affect you? Do you feel vulnerable?

You do not agree with a medical diagnosis expressed by another colleague of your patient. Do you feel incompetent?

You refuse in your operating room a female surgeon, starting from the idea that she is not capable and is not her place among? Is your gesture correct?

A patient asks you to stay and talk to him/ her after completing your visiting hours. What are you doing?

You refuse in your operating room a female surgeon, starting from the idea that she is not capable and is not her place among? Is your gesture correct?

As a resident doctor, you are told: “stay aside, do not touch but just watch”. Do you feel discriminated? What are you doing? How do you react?

You have scheduled an afternoon with your family only, but you are notified that you have an emergency. What are you choosing? Why?

At the hospital gate, the doorman legitimizes you. Do you think he has that right? Do you mind?

How do you feel when in the waiting room at the doctor, the nurse firsts let the married women enter the consultation and then the others. Do you mind? Why?

A gypsy mother comes to consultations with the child.

She took her number. It’s her turn. Do you take it by number, or do you let it wait after all?

On the bus you sit in a chair, and you are noticing that you are young. What are you doing?

You fall in love with a boy of a different ethnicity. You tell your parents? What are you doing? How do you solve the problem?

You fall in love with a girl of a different ethnicity. You tell your parents? What are you doing? How do you solve the problem?

A boy whistles you on the street. You turn?

What reaction do you have when, being a witness to a discussion, you hear: You these young people, you know nothing, you are not good for anything" ...

You revolt? Do you feel that they have prejudices?

You walk into a church and sit on a bench. Someone is warning you: This is not your sit. Get up!" What are you doing?

You're madly in love with your college who you happen to find out is a gypsy. Do you still love her?

You are a gypsy student and in the halls of the university a colleague calls you:

"Hey, gypsy, wait!" or "Hey, crows do not go in hot countries, are not traveling birds?" You, how are you, around here?" How do you react? What are you doing?

You are gypsy and you order a taxi. It’s coming, but the taxi driver when he sees you, immediately refuses the order. What are you doing? How react?

You walk into the mall next to a child who cries and claims he's lost. How react? You're taking him seriously?

At a wedding, folk music is played for all wedding guests (Romanians, Hungarians, Germans and gypsies). You are invited to a ceardaş (a traditional Hungarian dance). What are you doing? You refuse?

A gypsy asks you to take the seat free from your table. What are you doing?

On the bus in the free seat next to you, sit a gypsy, you get up? You're pulling? Do you mind?

In a local, at your table, sit a gypsy. What are you doing? How react?

In a local, at your table, sit a gypsy. What are you doing? How react?

Describe one or more concrete to/ in which you were involved/ or witnessed an act of discrimination (When? / Where? / How? / With whom? Why?)

5. My own experience…

1) I also lived in the moment when….

2) I felt vulnerable when….

3) I felt excluded when:

4) It is fair to be discriminated against when:

5) I was in the minority and I felt bad when:

6) Acceptance came at the time when:

7) We are equal when:

8) I felt the prejudice of others when:

9) Write what you can say:

10) Write what you cannot say:

11) Express a positive appreciation:

12) Express a negative appreciation:

6. Don't forget...

So, together without discrimination

a) for:

- to be people

- to be better

- to enrich our cultural values

- to consider people, being and not objects

b) Knowing that we will be:

- Specialists of tomorrow who, we will implement conduct and behavioral attitude in an informed way, meant to make the medical act an equal and common good of all

- Always, the one who will stretch out a hand to others

c) Being able to become tolerant:

- informing us correctly, having openness to new and change

- Showing responsibility

- Accepting diversity NOT unity-understanding the message

- Putting the health and life of the patient above all else

- Starting with respect and finally getting to it.

Notes

C. Bibliography

1. Astărăstoae V, Gavrilovici C, Vicol M, Gerely D, Sandu J (2011) – Ethics and non-discrimination of vulnerable groups in the health system, Ed. Grv. Popa UMF, Iași

2. Burtea V (2002), Gypsies in the synchronicity and diachrony of contact populations. Ed Lumina Lex, București

3. Coelho P (2012) - The manuscript of Acra, Ed.Humanitas, Bucharest

4. Lăzărescu M (1994) - Clinical Psychology, Ed Helican, Timişoara.

5. Paşca M.D. (2013) - Together without discrimination…- pliant-UMF- Tg.Mureş

6. Tudose Fl (2003) - The horizons of medical psychology, Ed Helicon, Timişoara.

7. The prayer http://www.library.da.ea lui Maimonides/Kellogg/Bioethies/codes/Maimonides.htm

8.The oath of Hipocrates http://www.univermedcdgm.ro/ineg/cnt/jurHipocra te.htlm

9. Universal Declaration of Human Rights

10. Law on the Rights of Children 46/2003

11. Law 95/2006 on reform in the domain healths

12. Code of medical deontology -2005

13. Law no 202/2002 prohibition of any form discrimination in access to all levels of medical assistance

www.ingramcontent.com/pod-product-compliance
Lightning Source LLC
LaVergne TN
LVHW010452160826
845677LV00012B/2454

* 9 7 9 8 8 9 2 4 8 5 9 9 9 *